ARE YOU
BIG ENOUGH?

A Guide by: Lawrence L. Bertoniere

Table of Contents

Introduction

First let me say congratulations on taking your first steps into the wonderfully rewarding world of PE. Many men would like to increase the size, and conditioning of their penis, yet few are willing to take the first step, swallow their pride, and admit it to themselves. Even fewer realize there is something they can do to increase not only the size, but overall health of their penis. You may now count yourself among these lucky, chosen few as you are now reading this book. Welcome to PE.

This book is intended as a gateway, a starting point, a true beginner's guide. This book will not attempt to turn you into a seasoned vet overnight, but instead be a gentle push in the correct direction. This book will outline some of the basic ideas, and theories required for proper understanding, and execution of a solid PE routine. You will be supplied with entry and intermediate work outs, suggested schedules and warning signs of improper technique.

Now, enough with the pleasantries. A bright new world awaits you.

What is PE?

PE can have one of two meanings for the sake of this book. PE can stand for either Penis Enlargement or Penis Exercise. While both can be taken to mean the same thing, they could also be used individually to better describe your desired results.

PE standing for Penis Enlargement

If you're here seeking only to increase the size of your penis, than you would most likely define PE as Penis Enlargement. The ultimate goal of most men who preform PE is a increase in the size of their penis.

PE standing for Penis Exercise

PE can also stand for Penis Exercise. If you are coming to PE seeking to increase the hardness of your erection, last longer in bed, or enhance your own sexual pleasure, than you would likely define PE as Penis Exercise.

What can I expect from PE?

Through following a solid and well-planned PE regimen, you can expect the benefits of both definitions of PE. You will not only achieve a larger penis but also a much healthier penis.

Physiologic indicators (PIs)

Physiologic indicators, from now on referred to as PIs, are positive, negative, or neutral feedback your penis gives you. By keeping an extremely close eye on your PIs, you're able to tell if your current PE workout is overworking your penis, underworking your penis or just right.

Clearly, overworking your penis is undesired. One does not simply jump into any workout going max force. Our bodies do not work this way. Over time, we slowly condition ourselves to the rigors of training. Only then are we able to push ourselves to higher extremes.

Underworking your penis, though not likely to cause problems, will result in little, if any gains. This is counterproductive; no one wants to put in months of hard work and effort with little or nothing to show for it.

The sweet spot: your penis should hang fuller, achieve erections easier, and over time, increase both length, and girth. This is, of course, the preferred response and clear indication of a well-planned, designed, and performed PE routine.

Types of PIs

Negative PIs are always signs of over training. If you experience pain, numbness, loss of size, you should reduce the time/force of your workouts.

Positive PIs clearly indicate you're on the correct path, your penis size has increased, it's hanging better, fuller, longer, your erections are stronger than they were before.

Neutral PIs are a little trickier. They, on their own, indicate neither negative nor positive results. To properly interpret Neutral PIs, you must take into consideration your other PIs.

If, for instance, you have been sticking to a well-planned and thought out PE workout for 2 weeks and you've noticed that your penis is very red after your routine, it hangs fuller though out the day, and you have been waking up with morning erections that would make a teenager jealous, it would be safe to say this is a Positive Neutral PI.

Two months later, you have increased your PE work out, you notice, after your daily PE routine, your penis has begun to have fluid buildup, a Neutral PI, unlike last time, your penis is no longer hanging fuller, and your morning erections have decreased, these are two clear Negative PIs, it is now safe to interpret your Neutral PI as a Negative, Neutral PI and it's clearly time to reduce your workload.

PIs list

Negative PIs

Pain or persistent discomfort

Reduced night and morning erections

Reduced hardness of erections

Discoloration

Loss of size that persists for more than a day

Positive PIs

Increased flaccid hang lasting all day

Increased night and morning erections

Increased hardness of erections

Increase of normal size

Increased or improved sexual desire

Neutral Pls

Short term contraction of penis after PE work out

Redness or spotting

Minor aches in your penis

Temporary increase in penis size

Fluid buildup; swelling under the penis skin

Loss of tug (LOT)

Loss of tug, from here on referred to as LOT, is a very basic PE concept with which you should become familiar. It is through knowing your LOT that you will learn how to better customize your length routine for maximum results.

LOT is of most use to those using devices for length gains. These are more strenuous forms of PE and therefore beyond the scope of this book. I would not suggest device usage to anyone just starting PE. However, everyone starting PE should take the time to figure out their LOT, since LOT is useful for determining how easily and quickly you will gain length.

The theory behind LOT is simple, those with high LOT: shorter, higher and tighter ligaments attached to their penis, have more potential for length gains than those with longer, lower, looser ligaments, i.e. low LOT. Shorter, higher and tighter ligaments will allow for maximum stretch before being limited by your penis' entry point into your body.

A low LOT should by no means deter you from PE. There have been those with extremely low LOTs who have made great progress, just as there have been others with very high LOTs that have had little or no gains. Do not look at LOT as a limiting factor. Instead, see it as a tool that will help maximize your results.

Determining LOT

Now that you understand why knowing your LOT is an important part of any beginners PE routine, it's time to learn how to find your LOT. Figuring out your LOT is a simple process, which turns off many would be PE'ers. Fear not, it's as simple as reading an analog clock.

To begin, you will need to hold the head of your penis with one of your hands, stretch your penis as far as possible without discomfort. Starting with your penis stretched up wards, facing your stomach, at 12 O'clock, contract your penis, you will feel your penis pull back. Pull back is what you are keeping track of and you should base this off feel, not sight.

Continue by moving your penis to the 11 O'clock position, 10 O'clock, and so on. You continue this process until you no longer physically feel your penis pull back. This is your LOT.

Most men start with a LOT of 6 – 8. Don't despair if you're a low lot, as mentioned earlier, LOT is a tool to improve your PE routine, not a rule set in stone.

Using LOT to maximize results

You now know your LOT, but how does this help you? LOT is used to figure out which angle, high or low, would be best to optimize your desired length gains.

Let's assume you went through the above steps, and learned you have a LOT of 9 O'clock. This would be considered a high LOT, in theory you have more potential for length gains than someone with a lower LOT. To take advantage of your higher LOT, you would want to focus on stretching the penis at lower angles, maximizing your ligament stretch.

Now, we'll assume you determined your LOT, and realized you have low LOT, 6 O'clock. A LOT of 6 would suggest you have less potential for gains at lower stretching angles, to maximize possible gains you would want to stretch at higher angles, facing upwards.

Regardless of your LOT, it is suggested you start stretching at lower angles, to max out possible ligament gains. To achieve the full benefits of ligament stretching you should attack all angles. Consider LOT a guide on where you should focus most but not all of your efforts.

Tunica

The tunica is the outer tissue that surrounds your penis' three corpus chambers and the smooth muscle within. The tunica acts much like a tire tube. It allows or limits the expansion of the inner smooth muscle. Once the max allowed expansion is reached, added pressure results in a harder erection instead of expansion.

Smooth muscle

A penis' smooth muscle determines its shape, size, and stiffness. When you're aroused, your smooth muscle is relaxed, allowing blood flow in. The relaxed smooth muscle expands as a result of blood being introduced, pushing against the tunica, trapping the blood within the smooth muscle.

Erection Quality (EQ)

Erection quality, from now on referred to as EQ, is the result of your smooth muscle filling or not filling your tunica. Stretching your tunica, without increasing your penis' smooth muscle will result in more possible tunica expansion but a much lower EQ.

The same idea applies to Increasing the amount of smooth muscle without stretching the tunica. Your EQ will improve greatly, giving you much harder erections, but you will not increase the girth of your penis, since the smooth muscles expansion is being limited by the tunica.

What does all this mean? How does it apply to me?

By understanding the two most important factors in determining your penis size and EQ, you can better focus on the desired results. There is little point in stretching your tunica if the underlining smooth muscle is already under-developed. There would also be no point in increasing your smooth muscle if your tunica is already a limiting factor, unless your goal is a harder penis.

The idea behind finding your limiting factor is to know which types of work outs to focus on. If you find that your penis isn't as hard as it was 10 years ago, then very likely your smooth muscle is the limiting factor. You would want to focus on exercises that expand the smooth muscle, pushing blood flow into your penis. You wouldn't be as worried about getting maximum stretch, as much as pushing the blood in and out.

If your penis is already rock hard, close to that of a teenager, then your tunica is likely the limiting factor. You would seek work outs that not only push blood into your penis, but also expanse the tunica as much as possible over extended times.

The most important part of any solid, safe PE routine is the warm up. This can't be stressed enough. Warming up not only increases your penis' ability to expand but also helps reduce the chance of injury. Don't overlook this key element to maximizing your PE goals, 15 minutes now can save you tons of heartache later.

Methods of warming up

There are several methods commonly used for pre-PE warm up. Some are excellent choices, others, not so much. The most commonly used methods are listed below.

Rice sock

This is by far the most reliable method, a simple sock, with ½ a cup of dry rice placed inside. Microwave for 30 – 45 seconds, shake up, check to insure it's an acceptable temperature, and then apply to the penis for 15 minutes.

Heating pad

Another tried and true method, heating pads are commonly used for pre-PE warm up. The main disadvantage of this method is the cord. You will have to find a spot close to an outlet and sit there for 15 minutes.

Warm wash cloth

A simple choice that most will have access to, simply wet, and microwave for 15 -30 seconds, check temperature, than apply for 15 minutes. The disadvantage to this approach is you will need to reheat the wash cloth several times over your warm up, best to prepare two or more.

The exercises

By now you should know what positive and negative warning signs to look out for, i.e., your PIs. You have figured out and understand your LOT. You now have a deeper understanding of what parts of your penis require work in order to increase girth and EQ. You have read about and plan to use one of the common methods of PE warm up. You have been set on the correct path to safely and knowledgeably start your PE journey.

There are countless forms of PE, they range from beginner to advanced to the insane! As stated earlier, this book will not attempt to address them all here. This book will detail the most common beginner and intermediate workouts. Just as in life, you have to crawl before you can walk, in PE you have to condition yourself before you attempt the more advanced exercises. It would be very careless and irresponsible of me to try and push a life time's worth of routines onto a beginner.

Below will be listed basic exercises you can use during your first year of PE with optimal results. Some you will carry with you through your entire PE experience. Others will be replaced with more advanced workouts later.

Let's get started, shall we?

Beginner PE routines

Beginner PE routines are just that, routines that are designed for someone just starting PE. This does not mean that they are without risk, in fact, it's just the opposite. You're more likely to get injured in your first 3 months of PE due to lack of conditioning and experience than someone who has months of proper PE training under their belt. That said, proceed with caution and never take undue risks.

Beginner PE routines: Stamina and EQ

The male kegel

The back bone of any solid PE routine, beginner or advanced, should be the male kegel. Not only does it help increase the overall EQ of your penis, when done correctly, it will increase your ability to last longer in bed.

The male kegel, while not directly responsible for increasing the size of your penis, does have the effect of improving the blood flow, helping maintain a healthier prostate and can lead to multiple male orgasms. There is little reason for any man to not add kegeling to their usual health regimen.

What is the male kegel? How do I find my PC muscle?

The male kegel is an exercise which directly strengthens your pubococcygeus muscle, from here on referred to as PC muscle, along with several associated muscles. By strengthening your PC muscle, you'll reap the benefits of improved orgasm control, harder erections, stronger orgasms and a multitude of other health benefits.

In order to kegel, you will first have to find the muscles to contract. The next time you're urinating, stop mid-flow. The muscles required to do this is your PC muscle.

How do I kegel?

To kegel, you must contract your PC muscle. Hold the contraction for as long as possible. This should *not* be done while urinating.

If you are like many men, you may not be able to hold your initial kegel for very long. This is ok, it simply means you have a weak PC muscle and will benefit all the more from this exercise.

How often should I kegel?

Like other muscles, your PC muscle requires rest between proper workouts. You should only kegel every other day, to allow yourself proper healing time.

Suggested kegel routine

Start off doing 50 or so kegels every other day. Hold each kegel for up to five seconds. Don't worry if you're not able to hold them for more than a second or two. As with any work out, your ability to do more will come with time.

Add more, and longer kegels over time, break your kegel workout into sessions spread out over your day. With time and effort, you will find they come naturally. Kegels can be done anywhere and any time, so take advantage of it.

Edging

Much like kegels, edging should be part of any man's PE routine that wants to not only last longer in bed, but also improve their EQ.

What is edging?

Edging is simply masturbating, stopping right before you ejaculate. Once you no longer feel the need to ejaculate, continue masturbation.

Edging is stamina training for your penis.

What are the benefits of edging?

There are many advantages associated with edging. Not only does edging improve your ability to last longer in bed, edging also works the penis' inner smooth muscles, promoting a healthier, stronger erection.

How do I edge?

You should start off your edging session with a well lubed erection. Masturbate until you feel the need to ejaculate, slowly reduce intensity.

Continue the above process until you can no longer hold back. Preferably twenty minutes, but, ten minutes should work well in the beginning.

Jelqing

Jelqing is the bread and butter size exercise of PE. If given the choice of one general exercise to do for the rest of your PE career, for not only size, but also EQ gains, your choice should be Jelqing.

Jelqing not only increases the length of your penis, but also the girth. Through Jelqing, you will push blood in and out of your penis, stretching the attached ligaments, expanding the tunica, working the underlining smooth muscles, and increasing the blood capacity of your veins.

You will carry this exercise with you throughout your entire PE career. Jelqing can not and should not be replaced.

Jelqing warning

Jelqing is widely considered the single most beneficial PE exercise that anyone, beginner or advanced, can perform. Jelqing is also one of the most dangerous, since it's generally one of the first exercises someone new to PE will add to their routine. If you are going to have early PE related injuries, Jelqing will likely be the cause. Below are several do's and don'ts of Jelqing.

Don't

Jelq without warming up first.

Dry Jelq, you should always Jelq well lubed.

Jelq at 100% erection.

Jelq over your glans/penis head, stop before you reach the head of your penis.

Apply max force, do not squeeze as hard as you can.

Do

Warm up before Jelqing.

Jelq well lubed.

Jelq at 40 - 75% erection level.

Stop before reaching your glans/penis head.

Lightly apply pressure.

What is Jelqing? What is the OK-grip?

Jelqing is a PE exercise that requires you to make an OK-grip, and milk your penis from its base, upwards to the base of the glans. Once again, never Jelq over your penis head.

The OK-grip is achieved by using your thumb, and index finger, to form an oval. Think of the 'ok' hand gesture. Overlap your index finger with your thumb as needed to form a tight, yet comfortable grip around your penis base. Make sure not to apply excessive force.

How do I Jelq?

You should take the time to understand and master Jelqing. Jelqing is as simple as making an OK-grip, and milking your penis. Jelqing, like all other PE exercises, can be extremely beneficial when done correctly. Jelqing can also cause permanent injury and penis deformation if done improperly. It is important you understand this before

continuing. Jelqing with poor technique can cause permanent erectile dysfunction!

Jelqing step by step

1. Apply lubrication to your penis.

2. Achieve an erection level of 40 – 75%.

3. Create an OK-grip with either hand around the base of your penis.

4. Lightly apply pressure to the OK-grip, slowly move from the base of your penis, to right under your penis glans/head. This should not hurt, but should

move blood though your penis. One Jelq should take 2 – 3 seconds.

5. Hold the OK-grip at the base of your glans, take your other hand and repeat process 3 - 4, letting go of your previous grip before starting the upward motion.

The idea here is a milking motion, one hand holding your penis in place, while the other is forming the OK-grip and milking your penis.

V-Jelq

The V-Jelq is a spinoff of the Jelq. The V-Jelq is useful for adding not only length, but also penis width.

All of the same warnings given for the Jelq apply to the V-Jelq. Though not considered an essential exercise, those wanting a more complete PE work out should add V-Jelq to their routine.

How do I V-Jelq?

The V-Jelq is much like the normal Jelq, but instead of an OK-grip, you use your index, and middle finger to make a peace sign.

Face your peace sign downwards, towards your legs. Face the palm of your peace signed hand towards your stomach, place your penis between your index and middle finger. Using your other hand, grasp the head of your penis. Starting from the base of your penis, work your stomach facing peace sign towards your penis glans/head. Once your peace sign hand reaches under your penis head, hold there, while you repeat the process with your other hand. Like the normal Jelq, never V-Jelq over your penis glans/head.

Penis stretching

Penis stretches are not only a good way to help warm your penis up for more intensive PE exercises, but is also instrumental in adding desired penis length.

Penis stretches can be done standing up or sitting down. You should only stretch your penis in a flaccid state for the first 6 months. You should stretch your penis before doing any workout that requires lubrication to avoid slippage.

How do I do penis stretches?

1. Hold your penis behind the head and softly pull straight out. Hold this position for 25 – 30 seconds.

2. Repeat the above step in four other directions. Left, down, right, up. Holding each stretch for 25 – 30 seconds.

You should apply enough force to stretch your penis' tissues but not hard enough to feel pain. It's best at first to apply too little force, then too much. As you become more conditioned to penis stretches, you can apply more force.

The most important part of penis stretching and any PE is that you don't feel pain. If at any time you feel a painful sensation, decrease the applied force.

Intermediate PE routines

Intermediate PE routines are generally reserved for those who have at least 2 – 3 months of regular PE experience under their belt. It is not suggested that you attempt any of these exercises without first being properly conditioned.

Intermediate PE routines: Girth

Flaccid Bend

The Flaccid Bend will most likely be one of the first intermediate girth exercises you will add to your workout. The Flaccid Bend is a backbone exercise for those seeking a thicker penis. You should not attempt to add Flaccid Bends to your workout until you've had at least six weeks of previous PE experience.

How do I do a Flaccid Bend?

Flaccid Bends require the use of two hands, using two or more fingers. One hand is used to grip the penis under the head while the other hand uses two or more fingers placed under the penis. The hand holding the penis head then bends the penis over the other hands fingers, holding for twenty to thirty seconds.

Flaccid Bends step by step

1. Start with an erection level of 30 – 60%.

2. Use one hand to grip your penis below its head, the same as if you were going to stretch.

3. Use your other hand to place two fingers underneath your penis.

4. Bend your penis over your two fingers.

5. Hold the bend for twenty to thirty seconds, avoiding any pain.

Now repeat the above steps in all directions. You will want to bend to the left, down, right, and up.

If you like, you can repeat the exercise by adding one finger each time, to a maximum of 4 fingers.

Side Jelq

The side Jelq is another extension of normal Jelqing. The side Jelq is considered an intermediate workout, and shouldn't be attempted without 3 months of PE experience.

Side Jelq step by step

1. Start with an erection level of 60 – 85%.

2. Began a normal Jelq. Half way through the Jelq, place your other hand at base of your penis. Your other hand will act as a support.

3. Curve your Jelq to the side.

4. As soon as your Jelq reaches the base of your penis head, press the palm of your hand at the base of your penis, against your penis shaft in a bending motion.

5. Repeat 15 – 20 times, alternating hands and sides.

Side to side stretches

Side to side stretches are an intermediate length gaining exercise. Side to side stretches should not be attempted until you have at least 3 months of PE experience.

Side to side stretches step by step

1. Your penis should be in a flaccid state for this exercise.

2. From a standing position grip your penis in either hand, thumbs up.

3. Pull your penis straight down, towards the floor.

4. While keeping pressure applied, slowly pull your penis to the left and then the right. This will count as one rep.

5. Repeat, doing 50 – 100 reps, starting from the middle each time.

Leg tuck pull

Another intermediate exercise for length and should not be attempted until you have 3 months of PE experience.

Leg tuck pull step by step

1. Your penis should be in a flaccid state for this exercise.

2. Laying on your back, grab your flaccid penis in your hand, thumb facing upwards.

3. Slowly stretch your penis downwards towards your feet.

4. Once you start to feel a good stretch, slowly raise your knees to your abdomen.

5. Do 15 – 25 reps.

Your beginners PE routine

So, now that you have access to several beginner and intermediate PE exercises, what's next? It's now time to set up a solid starter routine for you to follow.

The routine below is by no means your only possible choice. It is simply a PE work out plan that should work for most people. The below plan should be a starting point, something you can expand on with experience. If you feel that at some point you are over-working yourself with it, then do less. If you feel you're not getting enough out of it, then add more. Each person is unique, No one can custom tailor a routine that will work for everyone.

Your beginner PE routine

Week 1

Workout 1 day, take the next day off. 1 on, 1 off for the entire week.

Penis stretches, all 5 directions 25 seconds each.

Do 60 Jelqs, taking care not to apply to much force.

Do 25 kegels, holding for 1 – 5 seconds.

Pick one of your workout days to edge for 10 minutes.

Week 2

Workout 1 on, 1 off

Penis stretches, all 5 directions 25 seconds each.

Do 80 Jelqs, taking care not to apply to much force.

Do 30 kegels, holding for 1 – 5 seconds.

Pick one of your workout days to edge for 15 minutes.

Week 3

Workout 1 on, 1 off

Penis stretches, all 5 directions 30 seconds each.

Do 80 Jelqs, taking care not to apply to much force.

Do 40 V-Jelqs.

Do 40 kegels, holding for 2 – 5 seconds.

Pick one of your workout days to edge for 20 minutes.

Week 4

Workout 1 on, 1 off

Penis stretches, all 5 directions 30 seconds each.

Do 80 Jelqs, taking care not to apply to much force.

Do 60 V-Jelqs.

Do 50 kegels, holding for 3 – 5 seconds.

Pick two of your workout days to edge for 20 minutes.

Week 5

Workout 1 on, 1 off

Penis stretches, all 5 directions 30 seconds each.

Do 100 Jelqs, taking care not to apply to much force.

Do 80 V-Jelqs.

Do 50 kegels, Try holding for 5 seconds or more.

Pick two of your workout days to edge for 20 minutes.

Week 6

Workout 1 on, 1 off

Penis stretches, all 5 directions 30 seconds each.

Do 100 Jelqs, taking care not to apply to much force.

Do 100 V-Jelqs.

Do 50 kegels, Try holding for 5 seconds or more.

Pick two of your workout days to edge for 20 minutes.

Hopefully by week 6 you should have a good feeling for what you can, and can't handle. Be sure to watch your Pis. If at any point they are negative, reduce your workout, or take some time off. A week taken off by choice is preferred to being forced to take a month or more off due to injury. Try adding flaccid bends to your work out next week.

Supplements

No book on PE would be complete without suggesting supplements to help improve your PE gains. This is not an attempt to make a complete list of all available supplements, since that would take a full book just to scratch the surface. Below is listed a few of the more common supplements and their supposed use.

Ginkgo Biloba

Ginkgo Biloba is from a tree found in China. Ginkgo Biloba has long been cultivated for its ability to not only enhance memory, but improve blood flow. It is often taken as a means to offset Alzheimer's, or improve blood flow to all parts of the body. The use of Ginkgo has been found to improve the EQ of many men who take it. Ginkgo Biloba can be found at most major retail stores that sell supplements, at a cost of 10 dollars for a 3 month supply. It is suggested you take 60 – 200 mg a day, for best results.

Horny Goat Weed

Horny Goat Weed is a plant found in southern China and parts of Europe. Horny Goat Weed has long been considered an aphrodisiac, increasing the libido in both men and women. Supposed benefits of use include reduced general fatigue, improved erectile function and alleviation of menopausal discomfort. Horny Goat Weed, while not as affordable as Ginkgo Biloba, can still be a strong tool in any man's PE regimen who is attempting to get back the sexual vigor of his youth.

L-Arginine

L-Arginine is a chemical building block called "an amino acid" and is necessary for the body to make proteins. L-Arginine is found in red meats, fish, dairy products and poultry. L-Arginine helps with general blood flow, and therefore, can improve your EQ.

Penis enlargement pills

Penis enlargement pills work by improving the blood flow to your penis. As you age, the blood flow to your penis and other parts of your body is reduced, resulting in lower EQ. Reduction in EQ results in a smaller, erect penis. By increasing the blood flow to your penis, penis enlargement pills indirectly increase the size of your erection. The above mentioned supplements work in much the same way, and in most cases are much cheaper than penis enlargement pills. Proper PE training has the same affect, slowly improving the blood flow to your penis.

Green Tea

Not to be overlooked, Green tea has long been valued for its erection enhancing properties. Daily intake of Green tea is suggested for anyone hoping to improve the blood flow to their penis. Below is a recipe that should cause a temporary increase in the hardness of your erection by 10%.

Erection enhancing green tea

Bring four cups of water to a boil.

Add 4 – 5 bags of green tea.

Add 3 – 4 tablespoons of ground ginger.

Boil tea to desired strength.

Remove from heat, add in lemon and lime juice.

Sweeten with honey.

Reasons for the added ingredients?

Green tea is considered a cortisol blocker, which lowers your blood pressure.

Ginger has many of the same properties as Ginko Biloba and green tea.

Lemon and lime, naturally declog arteries.

Honey is know to raise testosterone levels.

Good luck

You have now been given all the necessary tools to began your PE journey. With the information you have learned from this book, you should be able to develop and follow a well-planned PE routine, customized to your needs.

Hopefully, you will look back on this book as the single most important investment of your life. A point and time where you said, I want more!

Good luck, in all your endeavors.

Warning

The author of this book is not a medical professional. The theories and ideas presented here have not been studied, or deemed safe by any medical professional or institution. You will apply any knowledge gained from this book at your own risk. You've been warned!

The information in this book is not intended for those under the age of 18.

www.ingramcontent.com/pod-product-compliance
Lightning Source LLC
Chambersburg PA
CBHW070458290526
45790CB00003B/1007